A GUIDE TO DEALING WITH

GRIEF

How to Heal and Find Strength While Grieving

Finlay Porter

Table of Contents

CHAPTER ONE: Introduction

Definition of Grief

Grief is a complex and multifaceted emotional response to loss. It encompasses a range of feelings such as sadness, despair, anger, confusion, and longing, often accompanied by physical sensations like fatigue or tightness in the chest. Grief can be triggered by various types of loss, including the death of a loved one, the end of a significant relationship, the loss of a job, or a significant change in one's life circumstances. It's a natural and necessary process that allows individuals to come to terms with their loss, adjust to a new reality, and eventually find meaning and hope again.

Importance of Understanding and Addressing Grief

It's important to recognise and deal with grief for several reasons:

1. **Mental and emotional well-being:** Unresolved grief can lead to prolonged emotional suffering, depression, anxiety, and other mental health issues. By understanding grief

and addressing it effectively, individuals can promote their own mental and emotional well-being.

2. **Physical health:** Grief can manifest physically, leading to symptoms such as fatigue, insomnia, changes in appetite, and even increased susceptibility to illness. Addressing grief can help mitigate these physical symptoms and promote overall health.

3. **Relationships:** Grief can strain relationships with friends, family, and colleagues, as individuals may struggle to communicate their feelings or

withdraw from social interactions. Understanding grief can help people navigate these challenges and maintain healthy connections with others.

4. **Workplace productivity:** Grieving employees may experience decreased productivity, difficulty concentrating, and absenteeism. Employers who understand and support employees through the grieving process can help maintain productivity and morale in the workplace.

5. **Preventing   complications:**
Unresolved grief can sometimes lead to complicated grief, a condition characterised by intense and prolonged symptoms that interfere with daily functioning. Addressing grief early on can help prevent the development of complicated grief and its associated complications.

6. **Personal growth:** While grief is painful, it can also be a catalyst for personal growth and transformation. By understanding and working through grief, individuals can develop

resilience, gain insight into themselves, and find new meaning and purpose in life.

Maintaining healthy relationships, encouraging personal development and resilience, and promoting mental, emotional, and physical well-being all depend on understanding and resolving sorrow.

CHAPTER TWO: Understanding Grief

Exploring the Nature of Grief

Examining the various facets of grief, such as its emotional, cognitive, physical, and spiritual components, is necessary to understand its nature. A summary of each is provided below:

1. **Emotional**: Grief encompasses a wide range of emotions, including sadness, anger, guilt, anxiety, loneliness, and numbness. These emotions may fluctuate in intensity

and can be triggered by various reminders of the loss. Understanding the emotional landscape of grief involves acknowledging and accepting these feelings as natural responses to loss.

2. **Cognitive**: Grief can affect cognitive functioning, leading to difficulties with concentration, memory, and decision-making. It may also involve intrusive thoughts or preoccupation with memories of the deceased. Exploring the cognitive aspects of grief involves recognising how loss impacts

thought processes and finding strategies to cope with cognitive challenges.

3. **Physical**: Grief is not just an emotional experience but also a physical one. It can manifest in physical symptoms such as fatigue, insomnia, loss of appetite, headaches, and muscle tension. Exploring the physical manifestations of grief involves understanding the mind-body connection and addressing physical symptoms through self-care practices and relaxation techniques.

4. **Spiritual**: For many people, grief raises existential questions and challenges their beliefs or sense of meaning in life. Exploring the spiritual dimension of grief involves grappling with issues of faith, mortality, and the afterlife. It may also involve finding solace and connection through rituals, prayer, or spiritual practices.

5. **Social**: Grief often impacts social relationships, as individuals may withdraw from others, struggle to communicate their feelings, or experience changes in their social

support network. Exploring the social aspects of grief involves understanding how loss affects relationships and finding ways to navigate interpersonal dynamics during the grieving process.

6. **Developmental**: Grief is a dynamic process that evolves and may be influenced by various factors, including the nature of the loss, the individual's coping resources, and their cultural and developmental context. Exploring the developmental aspects of grief involves recognising

that grief unfolds differently for each person and that there is no "right" way to grieve.

7. **Meaning-making**: Ultimately, exploring the nature of grief involves finding meaning and purpose amid loss. This may involve making sense of the loss, finding ways to honour the memory of the deceased, or discovering new sources of meaning and resilience. It is an ongoing process of adaptation and growth that continues long after the initial loss.

Common Misconceptions about Grief

Several common misconceptions surround grief, which can hinder understanding and empathy for those experiencing it. Here are a few:

1. **Grief has a timeline**: One of the most prevalent misconceptions is that grief follows a linear timeline and should resolve within a certain period. In reality, grief is a highly individualised process that varies in duration and intensity for each person. There is no "normal" timeline

for grieving, and it's essential to allow individuals to grieve at their own pace.

2. **Grief is solely emotional**: While grief is certainly emotional, it also encompasses physical, cognitive, and spiritual aspects. Many people experience physical symptoms such as fatigue, insomnia, or changes in appetite, as well as cognitive challenges like difficulty concentrating or making decisions. Recognising the multidimensional nature of grief is crucial for providing comprehensive support.

3. **Grief should be kept private**: Some individuals may feel pressure to keep their grief private or "put on a brave face" for others. However, grieving openly and seeking support from friends, family, or professionals can be essential for healing. Encouraging open communication about grief helps reduce stigma and fosters a supportive environment for those who are grieving.

4. **Grief should be "fixed" or "cured"**: There's a misconception that grief is something to be fixed or

cured, rather than something to be experienced and integrated into one's life. While grief may become more manageable over time, it doesn't necessarily go away completely. Instead, individuals learn to adapt to their loss and find ways to live with their grief.

5. **Grief follows a predictable pattern**: Another common misconception is that grief follows a predictable pattern or stages, such as the widely-known Kübler-Ross model of denial, anger, bargaining,

depression, and acceptance. While these stages may resonate with some people, they don't apply universally, and many individuals experience grief more fluidly and unpredictably.

6. **Grieving means forgetting**: Some people fear that grieving or moving forward means forgetting about the person they've lost. However, grieving doesn't mean forgetting; it's about finding ways to remember and honour the memory of the deceased while also finding a new way to live without them.

7. **Only death causes grief**: While death is a significant trigger for grief, it's not the only cause. Grief can result from any significant loss, including the end of a relationship, the loss of a job, a change in health status, or a major life transition. Recognising that grief can stem from various types of losses helps broaden our understanding and support for those who are grieving.

Different Types of Grief (e.g., anticipatory grief, disenfranchised grief)

Depending on the specifics of each situation and the type of loss experienced, grief can take many different forms. Among the typical forms of grieving are:

1. **Anticipatory grief**: This type of grief occurs before a significant loss, such as when a loved one is terminally ill or facing a life-threatening situation. Anticipatory grief allows individuals to begin the mourning process before the

actual loss occurs, but it can still be intense and challenging.

2. **Normal grief**: Normal grief is the typical response to a loss, such as the death of a loved one, the end of a relationship, or another significant life change. It involves a range of emotions and may include periods of sadness, anger, disbelief, and acceptance.

3. **Complicated grief**: Also known as prolonged or unresolved grief, complicated grief occurs when an individual experiences intense and

prolonged symptoms of grief that interfere with daily functioning. These symptoms may persist for an extended period, making it difficult for the individual to adjust to life without the deceased or to find meaning and purpose again.

4. **Disenfranchised   grief**: Disenfranchised grief refers to a loss that is not openly acknowledged or socially validated, such as the death of a pet, a miscarriage, or the loss of a job.   Individuals   experiencing disenfranchised grief may feel

unsupported or misunderstood by others, which can complicate the grieving process.

5. **Collective grief**: Collective grief occurs when a community or society experiences a shared loss, such as a natural disaster, a mass shooting, or a public tragedy. In these situations, individuals may grieve not only for their losses but also for the broader impact on their community or society as a whole.

6. **Ambiguous grief**: Ambiguous grief occurs when the circumstances

surrounding a loss are unclear or uncertain, such as when a loved one goes missing or is estranged from the family. In these situations, individuals may experience conflicting emotions and struggle to find closure or resolution.

7. **Secondary or vicarious grief**: Secondary grief refers to the grief experienced by individuals who are indirectly affected by a loss, such as friends, extended family members, or caregivers. Vicarious grief, on the other hand, occurs when individuals

experience grief in response to the loss experienced by someone else, such as when a therapist mourns the death of a client.

Knowing the many forms of grief can help people and communities cope with their own experiences of loss with empathy and compassion, as well as assist those who are grieving.

The Grieving Process: Stages and Dynamics

The grieving process is often conceptualised as having stages, though it's important to note that not everyone experiences these stages linearly or predictably. Here are commonly recognised stages of grief, along with some dynamics that may accompany them:

1. **Denial**: Initially, individuals may struggle to accept the reality of the loss. They may feel disbelief or numbness, finding it difficult to comprehend what has happened. Denial serves as a protective mechanism, shielding individuals from overwhelming emotions until they are ready to face reality.

2. **Anger**: As the reality of the loss sets in, individuals may experience intense feelings of anger. This anger can be directed towards various targets, including the deceased, oneself, other people, or even a higher power. It's a natural response to feeling helpless and out of control.

3. **Bargaining**: In an attempt to regain a sense of control or postpone the pain of loss, individuals may engage in bargaining. This can involve making deals with a higher power, such as praying for the return of the deceased

or promising to change certain behaviours in exchange for a different outcome. Bargaining reflects the desire to find meaning and make sense of the loss.

4. **Depression**: As the full weight of the loss sinks in, individuals may experience profound sadness and despair. This stage is characterised by feelings of emptiness, hopelessness, and a lack of interest in previously enjoyable activities. Depression is a natural response to the profound

sense of loss and the disruption of one's life.

5. **Acceptance**: Eventually, individuals come to accept the reality of the loss and begin to integrate it into their lives. Acceptance doesn't mean that the pain of grief disappears entirely, but rather that individuals can find a sense of peace and resolution. They may start to adjust to life without the deceased and find ways to remember and honour their memory.

These stages of grief are not necessarily sequential, and individuals may move back and forth between them, or experience them in a different order. Additionally, not everyone will experience all of these stages, and some may experience additional emotions or stages not listed here. The grieving process is highly individualised and influenced by factors such as the nature of the loss, the individual's personality, coping mechanisms, and support system.

CHAPTER THREE: Coping Mechanisms

Self-care Practices for Managing Grief

During the mourning process, self-care techniques are essential for fostering general wellbeing and managing bereavement. The following are some self-care techniques that anyone can use:

1. **Prioritise physical health**: Taking care of one's physical health can help manage the physical symptoms of grief and improve overall well-being. This includes getting regular exercise,

eating nutritious meals, staying hydrated, and getting enough sleep.

2. **Practice relaxation techniques**: Engaging in relaxation techniques such as deep breathing, meditation, yoga, or progressive muscle relaxation can help reduce stress and promote a sense of calmness and inner peace.

3. **Connect with others**: Seek support from friends, family, or support groups who can provide emotional support and understanding during difficult times. Talking about feelings and experiences with trusted

individuals can be healing and validating.

4. **Set boundaries**: It's important to set boundaries and prioritise self-care during the grieving process. This may involve saying no to additional responsibilities or commitments that feel overwhelming and allowing oneself time and space to grieve.

5. **Engage in activities that bring joy**: While grieving, it's important to engage in activities that bring joy, pleasure, and a sense of normalcy. This could include hobbies, spending

time in nature, listening to music, or engaging in creative expression.

6. **Practice self-compassion**: Be gentle and kind to yourself during the grieving process. Recognize that grieving is a natural and necessary response to loss and that it's okay to experience a range of emotions. Treat oneself with the same kindness and understanding that you would offer to a friend in a similar situation.

7. **Seek professional support**: Consider seeking support from a therapist, counsellor, or grief support

group if needed. Professional support can provide additional guidance, validation, and coping strategies for navigating the complexities of grief.

8. **Maintain routines**: While grieving, maintaining some sense of routine can provide stability and structure during a time of upheaval. This could include sticking to regular meal times, sleep schedules, or daily rituals.

9. **Express feelings**: Find healthy ways to express and process feelings of grief, whether through journaling, art, music, or talking with a trusted

confidant. Expressing emotions can help release pent-up feelings and promote healing.

10. **Practise patience and self-compassion**: Remember that healing from grief takes time, and it's important to be patient with oneself. Allow oneself to feel whatever emotions arise without judgement and trust that healing will come in its own time.

Healthy Coping Strategies

Coping with grief can be incredibly challenging, but several healthy strategies can help you navigate through the process:

1. **Allow Yourself to Feel**: It's important to acknowledge and accept your feelings, whether it's sadness, anger, guilt, or any other emotion. Allow yourself to experience these emotions without judgement..

2. **Seek Support**: Reach out to friends, family members, or a support group who can offer comfort and understanding. Talking about your

feelings with others who have experienced similar losses can be very therapeutic.

3. **Take Care of Yourself**: Make self-care a priority. Eat nutritious meals, get regular exercise, and try to get enough sleep. Taking care of your physical health can help you better cope with your emotional pain.

4. **Express Yourself**: Find healthy ways to express your feelings, such as journaling, art, music, or physical activity. Expressing yourself creatively can be a powerful outlet for grief.

5. **Practice Mindfulness**: Mindfulness techniques, such as deep breathing, meditation, or yoga, can help you stay grounded and present in the moment, reducing feelings of anxiety and overwhelm.

6. **Maintain Routine**: Stick to a routine as much as possible. Maintaining structure in your daily life can provide a sense of stability and control during a time of upheaval.

7. **Seek Professional Help if Needed**: If you're struggling to cope with your grief, don't hesitate to seek

help from a therapist or counsellor. They can provide support, guidance, and coping strategies tailored to your individual needs.

8. **Engage in Activities that Bring Comfort**: Engage in activities that bring you comfort and joy, whether it's spending time in nature, reading a good book, or engaging in a hobby you love.

9. **Be Patient with Yourself**: Grieving is a process that takes time, and it's okay to feel ups and downs along the way. Be patient and compassionate

with yourself as you navigate through your grief journey.

10. **Memorialise and Honour the Deceased**: Make a memorial, take part in a ritual or ceremony, or preserve their memory by telling stories and sharing happy memories with others are all methods to commemorate the memory of your loved one.

CHAPTER FOUR: Navigating Loss in Different Contexts

Loss of a Loved One

Dealing with the death of a family member or friend: Dealing with the death of a family member or friend is one of life's most difficult challenges. Here are some specific steps you can take to cope with the loss:

- **Allow Yourself to Grieve**: It's important to permit yourself to grieve in your way and at your own pace. There is no right or wrong way to grieve, and everyone experiences loss differently.

- **Reach Out for Support**: Lean on friends, family members, or a support group for comfort and understanding. Sharing your feelings with others who are also grieving can help you feel less alone.

- **Take Care of Yourself**: Make self-care a priority during this difficult time. Try to eat nutritious meals, get enough sleep, and engage in activities that bring you comfort and solace.

- **Express Your Feelings**: Find healthy ways to express your emotions, whether it's through talking, writing, art, music, or physical activity. Expressing your feelings can help you process your grief and find healing.

- **Memorialise Your Loved One**: Find meaningful ways to honour the memory of your loved one, such as creating a memorial, participating in a ritual or ceremony, or planting a tree in their honour.

- **Seek Professional Help if Needed**: If you're struggling to cope with your grief, don't hesitate to seek help from a therapist or counsellor. They can provide support, guidance, and coping strategies tailored to your individual needs.

- **Take One Day at a Time**: Grief is a process that takes time, and it's important to be patient with yourself as you navigate through it. Take each day as it comes and focus on taking small steps forward.

- **Find Meaning and Purpose**: Seek ways to find meaning and purpose in your life despite the loss. This could involve volunteering, pursuing a hobby or interest, or finding ways to honour your loved one's legacy.

- **Remember to Celebrate Their Life**: Instead of focusing solely on the loss, try to remember and celebrate the life of your loved one. Share stories, look at photos, and cherish the memories you shared.

- **Know That Healing Takes Time**: Healing from the death of a family member or friend is a gradual process, and it's normal to experience ups and downs along the way. Be patient with yourself and allow yourself the time you need to heal.

Supporting children through grief: Providing children with bereavement support necessitates a kind and perceptive approach. The following are some methods to assist kids in adjusting to the loss of a friend or family member:

- **Be Honest and Age-Appropriate**: Use clear and simple language to explain death to children, taking into account their age and level of understanding. Avoid using euphemisms like "gone to sleep" or "lost," as they can be confusing or frightening. Be honest about what has happened in a way that they can comprehend.

- **Encourage Expression of Feelings**: Let children know that it's okay to feel sad, angry, confused, or scared. Encourage them to express their emotions through talking, drawing, writing, or other creative outlets. Validate their feelings and reassure them that it's normal to have a range of emotions during this time.

- **Provide Reassurance and Comfort**: Offer reassurance that they are loved and supported and that it's not their fault. Provide physical comfort through hugs, cuddles, and other forms of affection. Let them know that it's okay to ask questions and that you're there to listen and provide answers to the best of your ability.

- **Maintain Routine and Stability**: Try to maintain regular routines as much as possible to provide a sense of stability and security for the child. Consistency in daily activities such as meals, bedtime routines, and school schedules can help them feel grounded during a time of upheaval.

- **Encourage Memories and Remembrance**: Encourage children to share memories of the person who has died and participate in activities to honour their memory, such as creating a memory box, planting a tree, or writing a letter. Remind them that it's okay to talk about the person and keep their memory alive.

- **Provide Age-Appropriate Information**: Answer questions honestly and provide information about death in a way that is appropriate for the child's age and developmental stage. Avoid overwhelming them with too much information at once, but be prepared to provide additional explanations as they seek to understand.

- **Seek Professional Support if Needed**: If a child is struggling to cope with their grief or is experiencing prolonged distress, consider seeking support from a counsellor, therapist, or other mental health professional who specialises in working with children and grief.

- **Take Care of Yourself**: Supporting a grieving child can be emotionally taxing, so it's important to take care of yourself as well. Make sure to prioritise self-care and seek support from other adults or professionals if you need it.

By providing love, support, and understanding, you can help children navigate the grieving process healthily and constructively.

Coping with the loss of a pet: Losing a pet can be incredibly difficult, as they often become cherished members of our families. Here are some ways to cope with the loss:

- **Allow yourself to grieve:** Recognise that it's okay to feel sad, angry, or even guilty about the loss of your pet. Permit yourself to experience these emotions.

- **Share your feelings:** Talk to friends, family, or a therapist about your emotions. Sharing your feelings can provide comfort and support during this difficult time.

- **Create a tribute:** Consider creating a tribute to your pet, such as a photo album or a memory box filled with mementoes. This can help you honour their memory and provide a sense of closure.

- **Maintain routines:** Stick to your daily routines as much as possible. Maintaining a sense of normalcy can help provide stability during a time of grief.

- **Seek support:** Reach out to pet loss support groups or online forums where you can connect with others who have experienced similar losses. Sharing your experiences with others who understand can be incredibly comforting.

- **Take care of yourself:** Make sure to take care of your physical and emotional needs during this time. Eat well, get enough sleep, and engage in activities that bring you joy and comfort.

- **Memorialise your pet:** Consider holding a memorial service or planting a tree in your pet's honour. Doing something to memorialise your pet can provide a sense of closure and help you remember them fondly.

- **Consider adopting again:** While it may take time, consider opening your heart to another pet in the future. While no pet can replace the one you lost, opening your home to a new furry friend can bring joy and companionship back into your life.

Keep in mind that every person experiences grief differently, so it's critical to choose what method of grieving works best for you. Give yourself the time and space you need to heal, and remember that it's acceptable to ask for help when you need it.

Other Forms of Loss

Loss of a Job or Career: Losing a job or having a career setback can be extremely difficult and have a wide-ranging impact on your life. Here are some steps for dealing with this situation:

Allow yourself to grieve: Losing a job can bring about feelings of shock, anger, sadness, and even a sense of identity loss. It's important to acknowledge and accept these emotions rather than suppressing them.

Reach out for support: Lean on friends, family members, or a mentor for emotional support during this time. Talking about your feelings and receiving encouragement from others can help you feel less isolated and more hopeful about the future.

Take care of yourself: Focus on self-care activities such as exercising regularly, eating healthily, getting enough sleep, and practise relaxation techniques like meditation or deep breathing. Taking care of your physical and mental well-being is essential during times of stress.

Reflect on your strengths and accomplishments: Take some time to reflect on your past achievements and the skills you've developed throughout your career. Remind yourself of your value and the contributions you've made in your previous roles.

Set realistic goals: Assess your skills, interests, and career aspirations, and then set realistic short-term and long-term goals for yourself. Break down these goals into manageable steps, and create a plan to work towards them.

Update your resume and LinkedIn profile: Take this opportunity to update your resume, LinkedIn profile, and other professional materials. Highlight your skills, accomplishments, and experiences that are relevant to your desired career path.

Network: Reach out to former colleagues, mentors, and other professionals in your industry for networking opportunities. Attend industry events, join professional associations, and participate in online networking groups to expand your network and learn about potential job opportunities.

Consider new opportunities: Explore different career paths, industries, or job roles that align with your skills, interests, and values. Keep an open mind and be willing to adapt to new opportunities that may arise.

Seek additional education or training: Consider pursuing further education, certifications, or training programmes to enhance your skills and qualifications. Investing in your professional development can increase your marketability and open up new career opportunities.

Stay positive and resilient: Remember that setbacks are a natural part of life and can often lead to new opportunities for growth and development. Stay positive, resilient, and proactive in your job search efforts, and believe in your ability to overcome challenges and achieve success in your career.

Loss of Health or Independence: Losing one's freedom or health can be extremely difficult; however, there are strategies to deal with the changes and adjust:

1. **Seek Support**: Reach out to friends, family, or support groups who can offer emotional support and practical assistance. Having a strong support network can help you feel less isolated and more empowered to navigate through difficult times.

2. **Acceptance**: Acknowledge and accept the changes in your health or level of independence. While it's natural to feel a range of emotions,

including sadness, anger, or frustration, accepting your new reality can be the first step towards finding peace and making adjustments.

3. **Focus on What You Can Control**: Instead of dwelling on things you can't change, focus on what you can control. This might include making lifestyle adjustments, seeking medical treatment or therapy, or finding alternative ways to accomplish tasks.

4. **Adaptation and Flexibility**: Be willing to adapt and find new ways of doing things. This might involve using

assistive devices, modifying your living environment, or learning new skills to maintain independence.

5. **Maintain a Positive Outlook**: Cultivate a positive mindset and focus on the things that bring you joy and fulfilment. Practice gratitude for the things you still have and celebrate your achievements, no matter how small they may seem.

6. **Stay Active and Engaged**: Stay engaged in activities and hobbies that bring you joy and fulfilment. This can help boost your mood, maintain a

sense of purpose, and prevent feelings of isolation.

7. **Prioritise Self-Care**: Take care of your physical and mental well-being by prioritising self-care activities such as exercise, healthy eating, adequate sleep, and relaxation techniques like meditation or mindfulness.

8. **Advocate for Yourself**: Don't hesitate to advocate for your needs and rights. Communicate openly with healthcare providers, caregivers, and loved ones about your preferences, concerns, and goals for your care.

9. **Seek Professional Help**: If you're struggling to cope with the loss of health or independence, consider seeking professional help from a therapist or counsellor who specialises in dealing with these issues. Therapy can provide you with coping strategies, emotional support, and guidance on how to adjust to life changes.

10. **Stay Connected**: Stay connected with others and maintain social connections as much as possible. Whether it's through in-person visits,

phone calls, or video chats, staying connected with loved ones can provide comfort, support, and a sense of belonging.

Loss through Divorce or Relationship Breakup: Divorce and breakups can be emotionally taxing and cause feelings of loss, sadness, and uncertainty. Here are some strategies for handling this challenging circumstance:

1. **Allow Yourself to Grieve**: It's natural to feel a range of emotions, including sadness, anger, confusion,

and even relief. Allow yourself to experience these emotions without judgement and give yourself time to process the loss.

2. **Seek Support**: Lean on friends, family members, or a therapist for emotional support during this challenging time. Talking about your feelings and receiving validation and empathy from others can help ease the pain of the breakup.

3. **Take Care of Yourself**: Focus on self-care activities such as exercise, healthy eating, adequate sleep, and

relaxation techniques like meditation or yoga. Taking care of your physical and emotional well-being is essential for coping with the stress of a breakup.

4. **Create Boundaries**: Establish clear boundaries with your ex-partner to protect your emotional well-being and facilitate the healing process. This might include limiting contact, setting communication guidelines, or seeking the support of a mediator if necessary.

5. **Reflect on the Relationship**: Take some time to reflect on the relationship and identify any patterns,

behaviours, or issues that contributed to its demise. Use this opportunity for self-reflection and personal growth to learn from the experience and avoid making the same mistakes in future relationships.

6. **Focus on the Future**: Instead of dwelling on the past or what could have been, focus on the future and the opportunities it holds. Set new goals, pursue your passions, and envision the life you want to create for yourself moving forward.

7. **Stay Connected**: Surround yourself with supportive people who uplift and encourage you during this difficult time. Maintain social connections, participate in activities you enjoy, and seek out new opportunities for connection and growth.

8. **Seek Closure**: If possible, seek closure with your ex-partner by having an open and honest conversation about the breakup. Express your feelings, ask any lingering questions, and work towards finding resolution and closure.

9. **Seek Professional Help**: If you're struggling to cope with the emotional aftermath of a breakup, consider seeking professional help from a therapist or counsellor who specialises in relationship issues. Therapy can provide you with coping strategies, emotional support, and guidance on how to heal and move forward.

10. **Give Yourself Time**: Healing from a breakup takes time, so be patient with yourself and allow yourself to heal at your own pace. Remember that it's okay to feel sad,

angry, or lost, and that healing is a gradual process that unfolds over time.

CHAPTER FIVE: Finding Meaning and Purpose

The Search for Meaning in Grief

It is normal for people to look for meaning in their grief, and doing so might provide them some comfort and closure in the face of their loss's agony. Observe and discover purpose in your grief in the following ways:

1. **Reflect on Memories**: Reflect on the memories and experiences you shared with the person you've lost. Cherish the moments you had

together and find comfort in the love and connection you shared.

2. **Find Purpose in Pain**: Consider how your experience of grief can lead to personal growth and transformation. Use your grief as an opportunity to reflect on your values, priorities, and goals in life, and consider how you can live more fully and authentically in honour of your loved one.

3. **Seek Spiritual or Philosophical Perspectives**: Explore spiritual or philosophical perspectives on life,

death, and the nature of existence. Seek solace in beliefs or practices that provide comfort and meaning, whether it's through religion, spirituality, meditation, or mindfulness.

4. **Connect with Others**: Connect with others who have experienced similar losses and share your stories, thoughts, and feelings. Finding support and validation from others who understand your grief can help you feel less alone and find meaning in shared experiences.

5. **Channel Grief into Action**: Channel your grief into meaningful action by volunteering, advocating for causes you believe in, or participating in activities that honour the memory of your loved one. Finding ways to make a positive impact in the world can give your grief a sense of purpose and meaning.

6. **Express Your Emotions**: Allow yourself to express your emotions openly and honestly, whether it's through writing, art, music, or conversation. Expressing your feelings

can help you process your grief and find meaning in the depths of your pain.

7. **Find Comfort in Rituals and Traditions**: Participate in rituals or traditions that hold meaning for you and your loved one, whether it's lighting a candle in their memory, visiting their favourite place, or celebrating special occasions in their honour. These rituals can provide a sense of connection and continuity amidst the loss.

8. **Seek Professional Guidance**: If you're struggling to find meaning in your grief, consider seeking guidance from a therapist, counsellor, or grief support group. A trained professional can help you explore your feelings, beliefs, and experiences in a supportive and nonjudgmental environment.

Recall that there is no right or wrong way to travel the process of finding meaning in loss; it is a personal and unique experience. Recognise that healing requires time and self-compassion, and be patient and kind with yourself as you work through and make sense of your grief.

Transforming Grief into Growth

Transforming grief into growth is a powerful process that involves finding meaning, resilience, and personal development in the face of loss. Here are some ways to turn grief into an opportunity for growth:

1. **Acknowledge Your Feelings**: Allow yourself to fully experience and acknowledge your emotions, including sadness, anger, guilt, and fear. Embracing your feelings rather than

suppressing them is the first step toward healing and growth.

2. **Reflect on Your Values**: Use the experience of grief as an opportunity to reflect on your values, priorities, and goals in life. Consider what truly matters to you and how you want to live moving forward. Clarifying your values can help you align your actions with your deepest desires and aspirations.

3. **Seek Meaning**: Explore the meaning of your loss and how it fits into the larger context of your life story. Look

for lessons, insights, or silver linings that can emerge from the experience of grief. Finding meaning in your loss can provide a sense of purpose and direction as you navigate through the healing process.

4. **Practice Self-Compassion**: Be gentle and compassionate with yourself as you grieve. Treat yourself with kindness, understanding, and patience, and allow yourself the time and space to heal at your own pace. Self-compassion is essential for

building resilience and promoting growth in the face of adversity.

5. **Learn from the Experience**: Use the experience of grief as an opportunity for self-reflection and personal growth. Consider how the loss has impacted you, what you've learned about yourself and others, and how you can grow from the experience. Every challenge presents an opportunity for growth and self-discovery.

6. **Cultivate Resilience**: Cultivate resilience by developing coping skills,

practising gratitude, fostering social connections, and maintaining a positive outlook on life. Resilience is the ability to bounce back from adversity and thrive in the face of challenges, and it can be strengthened through practice and perseverance.

7. **Connect with Others**: Seek support from friends, family members, or support groups who can provide encouragement, empathy, and understanding as you navigate through grief. Connecting with others who have experienced similar losses

can remind you that you're not alone and that healing is possible.

8. **Channel Grief into Action**: Channel your grief into meaningful action by engaging in activities that honour the memory of your loved one or contribute to causes you believe in. Whether it's volunteering, advocating for change, or pursuing creative outlets, finding purpose in your grief can help you grow and find meaning amid loss.

9. **Embrace Growth Mindset**: Embrace a growth mindset, which

involves viewing challenges as opportunities for learning and growth. Instead of seeing grief as an obstacle, approach it as a chance to develop resilience, compassion, and wisdom. Adopting a growth mindset can help you navigate through grief with strength and optimism.

10. **Seek Professional Help**: If you're struggling to cope with grief or find meaning in your loss, consider seeking guidance from a therapist, counsellor, or grief support group. A trained professional can provide you

with tools, strategies, and support to facilitate your growth journey and help you navigate through the challenges of grief.

Honouring the Memory of the Deceased

Paying respect to a departed loved one's memory is a highly personal and meaningful approach to maintaining their spirit and finding solace during a period of bereavement. In commemoration of them, consider the following:

1. **Create a Memorial**: Consider creating a memorial or tribute in honour of your loved one. This could be a physical memorial such as a plaque, bench, or garden, or a digital memorial such as a website, social media page, or online memorial tribute.

2. **Celebrate Their Life**: Host a celebration of life ceremony or gathering to honour and remember your loved one. Invite friends and family to share stories, memories, and anecdotes about the deceased, and

create a space for reflection, connection, and healing.

3. **Share Their Legacy**: Share stories, photos, and mementoes of your loved one with others. Keep their memory alive by talking about them, sharing their accomplishments and values, and passing on their wisdom and teachings to future generations.

4. **Continue Their Traditions**: Carry on traditions, rituals, and customs that were meaningful to your loved one. Whether it's cooking their favourite meal, participating in their

favourite activities, or observing special holidays and anniversaries, continuing their traditions can help you feel connected to their memory.

5. **Create a Memory Book or Scrapbook**: Compile photos, letters, keepsakes, and other memorabilia in a memory book or scrapbook dedicated to your loved one. This can serve as a tangible reminder of their life and legacy, and provide comfort and solace during times of grief.

6. **Support a Cause**:Honour your loved one's memory by supporting a cause

or charity that was important to them. Whether it's donating, volunteering your time, or organising a fundraiser in their honour, supporting a cause can be a meaningful way to keep their spirit alive and make a positive impact in their memory.

7. **Create a Memorial Fund or Scholarship**: Establish a memorial fund or scholarship in your loved one's name to support causes or organisations that were important to them. This can provide a lasting legacy

and honour their passions, values, and contributions to the community.

8. **Perform Acts of Kindness**: Perform acts of kindness and generosity in honour of your loved one. Whether it's helping a neighbour in need, volunteering at a local charity, or performing random acts of kindness for strangers, spreading love and compassion can honour your loved one's memory and make the world a better place.

9. **Visit Their Final Resting Place**: Visit your loved one's final resting

place regularly to pay your respects and find solace in their presence. Take time to reflect, pray, or meditate, and find comfort in the peaceful surroundings.

10. **Keep Their Memory Alive in Your Heart**: Ultimately, the most important way to honour the memory of your loved one is to keep them alive in your heart and cherish the time you shared. Remember their love, laughter, and legacy, and carry their spirit with you as you navigate through life's journey.

Creating a Legacy of Love and Resilience

One of the most effective ways to make a lasting impression on the world and encourage others to live bravely, compassionately, and strongly is to leave a legacy of love and perseverance. The following are some methods for leaving such a legacy:

1. **Lead by Example**: Live your life with love, kindness, and resilience, and lead by example for others to follow. Show compassion towards others, overcome adversity with grace

and strength, and demonstrate resilience in the face of challenges.

2. **Practice Empathy and Understanding**: Cultivate empathy and understanding towards others by listening with an open heart, offering support and encouragement, and validating their experiences and emotions. Show compassion towards those who are struggling and extend a helping hand whenever possible.

3. **Be a Source of Support**: Be a source of support and encouragement for others who are facing adversity or

going through difficult times. Offer a listening ear, provide practical assistance, and offer words of wisdom and comfort to help them navigate through challenges with resilience and hope.

4. **Foster Connection and Community**: Build connections and foster a sense of community among family, friends, and neighbours. Create a supportive network where individuals can lean on each other for support, share their struggles and

triumphs, and find strength and resilience in the power of community.

5. **Share Your Story**: Share your own experiences of love and resilience with others to inspire and empower them on their journey. Be open and vulnerable about the challenges you've faced and the lessons you've learned, and offer hope and encouragement to those who may be struggling.

6. **Teach Life Skills**: Teach life skills and coping strategies that promote resilience and well-being, such as problem-solving, stress management,

self-care, and positive thinking. Empower others with the tools they need to navigate through life's challenges with strength and resilience.

7. **Support Causes and Charities**: Support causes and charities that promote love, compassion, and resilience in the world. Whether it's supporting organisations that provide aid to those in need, advocating for social justice and equality,or promoting mental health and well-being, find ways to make a

positive impact and leave a legacy of love and resilience.

8. **Create Meaningful Relationships**: Invest in meaningful relationships with family, friends, and loved ones based on love, trust, and mutual respect. Nurture these relationships with care and attention, and leave a lasting legacy of love and connection that transcends time and space.

9. **Celebrate Strength and Resilience**: Celebrate and honour acts of strength and resilience in

yourself and others. Acknowledge and celebrate the courage, perseverance, and resilience that individuals demonstrate in overcoming adversity and finding hope and healing during challenges.

10. **Pass on Your Values and Beliefs**: Pass on your values, beliefs, and life lessons to future generations. Share your wisdom, stories, and experiences with your children, grandchildren, and others, and inspire them to live with love, resilience, and compassion in their own lives.

CHAPTER SIX: Moving Forward

Embracing Life after Loss

It takes bravery to embrace life after loss, which entails discovering meaning, healing, and hope while grieving. Here are a few strategies for embracing life after loss:

1. **Allow Yourself to Grieve**: Give yourself permission to grieve and feel your emotions fully. It's normal to experience a range of emotions, including sadness, anger, guilt, and fear. Embracing your grief allows you

to process your feelings and begin the healing process.

2. **Seek Support**: Lean on friends, family, or a support group for emotional support during this difficult time. Talking about your feelings and sharing your experiences with others who understand can provide comfort and validation as you navigate through grief.

3. **Practice Self-Care**: Take care of your physical, emotional, and spiritual well-being by practising self-care activities such as exercise, healthy

eating, adequate sleep, and relaxation techniques like meditation or yoga. Prioritising self-care helps you build resilience and cope with the stress of loss.

4. **Find Meaning in Your Loss**: Look for meaning and purpose in your loss by reflecting on the lessons you've learned, the growth you've experienced, and how your loved one's memory continues to inspire you. Finding meaning in your loss can provide comfort and help you move forward with hope and resilience.

5. **Celebrate Your Loved One's Life**: Honour and celebrate the life of your loved one by sharing memories, stories, and anecdotes about them with others. Keep their memory alive by participating in activities they enjoyed, continuing their traditions, and supporting causes or charities that were important to them.

6. **Set Realistic Goals**: Set realistic goals for yourself and take small steps towards rebuilding your life after loss. Whether it's returning to work, pursuing hobbies and interests, or

reconnecting with friends and loved ones, setting goals gives you a sense of purpose and direction as you move forward.

7. **Stay Connected**: Stay connected with friends, family, and your support network as you navigate through grief. Surround yourself with people who uplift and support you, and seek out opportunities for social connection and meaningful relationships.

8. **Embrace New Opportunities**: Be open to new experiences, opportunities, and relationships that

come your way. Embracing life after loss means embracing the present moment and being willing to explore new paths and possibilities for growth and fulfilment.

9. **Practice Gratitude**: Cultivate a sense of gratitude for the blessings and opportunities in your life, even amidst the pain of loss. Focusing on the positive aspects of your life can help shift your perspective and foster resilience as you embrace life after loss.

10. **Seek Professional Help if Needed**: If you're struggling to cope with grief or find meaning in your loss, don't hesitate to seek professional help from a therapist, counsellor, or grief support group. A trained professional can provide you with tools, strategies, and support to navigate through the challenges of grief and embrace life with resilience and hope.

Adjusting to a New Normal

While readjusting to a new normal following a major loss or life transition can be difficult, it's a crucial step in the healing process. Here are some techniques to aid with your adjustment:

1. **Acknowledge the Change**: Recognise that your life has changed and that it's okay to feel a range of emotions, including sadness, anger, confusion, and even relief. Accepting the reality of the situation is the first step toward adjusting to your new normal.

2. **Give Yourself Time**: Be patient with yourself as you navigate through the adjustment process. Healing takes

time, and it's okay to take things one day at a time. Allow yourself to grieve and experience the full range of emotions associated with your loss or life change.

3. **Create Structure**: Establishing a new routine or structure can provide a sense of stability and predictability as you adjust to your new normal. Set regular daily routines for activities such as meals, exercise, work, and sleep to help you feel grounded and organised.

4. **Set Realistic Expectations**: Be realistic about what you can accomplish and what you need to prioritise during this time of adjustment. Set achievable goals for yourself and focus on taking small steps forward each day.

5. **Focus on Self-Care**: Take care of your physical, emotional, and mental well-being by prioritising self-care activities such as exercise, healthy eating, adequate sleep, and relaxation techniques like meditation or mindfulness. Taking care of yourself is

essential for coping with stress and building resilience.

6. **Stay Connected**: Stay connected with friends, family, and your support network as you navigate through your new normal. Lean on others for emotional support, encouragement, and practical assistance, and be willing to ask for help when you need it.

7. **Practice Flexibility and Adaptability**: Be open to adapting to changes and making adjustments as needed. Life is unpredictable, and

learning to be flexible and adaptable can help you navigate through unexpected challenges and transitions.

8. **Focus on the Positives**: Look for silver linings and opportunities for growth and learning in your new normal. Focus on the things you can control and the positive aspects of your life, rather than dwelling on what you've lost or what you can't change.

9. **Seek Meaning and Purpose**: Look for meaning and purpose in your new normal by exploring opportunities for personal growth, connection, and

contribution. Find activities, hobbies, or causes that bring you joy and fulfilment, and pursue them with passion and enthusiasm.

10. **Seek Professional Help if Needed**: If you're struggling to adjust to your new normal or experiencing significant distress, don't hesitate to seek professional help from a therapist, counsellor, or support group. A trained professional can provide you with guidance, support, and coping strategies to help you

navigate through this challenging time.

Setting Goals and Aspirations for the Future

Particularly after suffering a major loss or going through a large life transition, setting goals and objectives for the future is an empowering approach to going forward with purpose and direction. Here's how to make your objectives and dreams meaningful:

1. **Reflect on Your Values and Priorities**: Take some time to reflect on what matters most to you in life.

Consider your values, passions, and long-term aspirations. Your goals should align with these core values and reflect what you truly want to achieve.

2. **Identify Specific Goals**: Break down your aspirations into specific, measurable, achievable, relevant, and time-bound (SMART) goals. For example, instead of setting a vague goal like "get healthier," you might set a SMART goal like "exercise for 30 minutes five days a week" or "cook at least three healthy meals per week."

3. **Set Short-Term and Long-Term Goals**: Consider setting both short-term and long-term goals to give you a sense of direction and progression. Short-term goals can help you make progress quickly and build momentum, while long-term goals provide a vision for your future and motivate you to stay focused and committed.

4. **Break Goals into Actionable Steps**: Break down your goals into smaller, actionable steps that you can take to move closer to achieving them.

This makes your goals feel more manageable and increases your likelihood of success. Focus on taking consistent, incremental steps forward each day.

5. **Stay Flexible and Adaptive**: Be open to adjusting your goals and aspirations as needed based on changing circumstances, priorities, and opportunities. Life is unpredictable, and it's important to remain flexible and adaptive in pursuit of your goals.

6. **Visualise   Success**: Visualise yourself achieving your goals and living your aspirations. Imagine how it will feel when you accomplish what you set out to do. Visualisation can help you stay motivated and focused on your goals, even when faced with challenges or setbacks.

7. **Seek Support and Accountability**: Share your goals and aspirations with friends, family, or a mentor who can provide support, encouragement, and accountability. Having someone to cheer you on and hold you

accountable can help keep you motivated and on track.

8. **Celebrate Progress**: Celebrate your progress and achievements along the way, no matter how small. Acknowledge your hard work and perseverance, and take time to reward yourself for reaching milestones and making strides towards your goals.

9. **Stay Committed and Persistent**: Stay committed to your goals and aspirations, even when faced with obstacles or setbacks. Remember that setbacks are a natural part of the

journey, and persistence is key to overcoming challenges and achieving success.

10. **Review and Adjust Regularly**: Regularly review your goals and aspirations to track your progress and make any necessary adjustments. Reflect on what's working well and what could be improved, and make changes as needed to keep moving forward towards your vision for the future.

Maintaining Ongoing Self-care and Support Systems

Sustaining continuous self-care and support networks is essential, particularly during periods of transition or bereavement. The following techniques will assist you in making self-care a priority and creating a solid support system:

1. **Establish Daily Self-Care Rituals**: Incorporate self-care activities into your daily routine, such as meditation, exercise, journaling, reading, or spending time outdoors. Prioritise activities that help you relax, recharge,

and nourish your mind, body, and soul.

2. **Practice Mindfulness and Relaxation Techniques**: Practise mindfulness meditation, deep breathing exercises, or progressive muscle relaxation to help reduce stress, anxiety, and overwhelm. These techniques can help you stay grounded, present, and centred amidst life's challenges.

3. **Maintain Healthy Habits**: Prioritise your physical health by eating a balanced diet, getting regular

exercise, staying hydrated, and getting enough sleep. Taking care of your body can help boost your mood, energy levels, and overall well-being.

4. **Set Boundaries**: Establish healthy boundaries to protect your time, energy, and emotional well-being. Learn to say no to activities or commitments that drain you or don't align with your priorities, and prioritise activities that bring you joy and fulfilment.

5. **Seek Professional Help if Needed**: If you're struggling to cope

with stress, anxiety, depression, or grief, don't hesitate to seek support from a therapist, counsellor, or mental health professional. Therapy can provide you with tools, strategies, and support to navigate through difficult emotions and experiences.

6. **Stay Connected with Others**: Cultivate meaningful connections with friends, family, and your support network. Lean on others for emotional support, encouragement, and companionship, and be willing to offer support in return. Staying connected

with others can help you feel less alone and more resilient during challenging times.

7. **Join Support Groups**: Consider joining a support group or community for individuals who have experienced similar losses or life changes. Sharing your experiences, thoughts, and feelings with others who understand can provide validation, empathy, and a sense of belonging.

8. **Engage in Meaningful Activities**: Participate in activities that bring you joy, fulfilment, and a sense of purpose.

Whether it's pursuing hobbies, volunteering, or engaging in creative outlets, find activities that nourish your soul and help you connect with your passions and interests.

9. **Practice Self-Compassion**: Be kind and compassionate towards yourself, especially during times of stress or difficulty. Treat yourself with the same kindness and understanding that you would offer to a friend in need, and practice self-compassionate self-talk.

10. **Regularly Assess and Adjust**: Regularly assess your self-care

practices and support systems to ensure they're meeting your needs. Be willing to adjust your routines, habits, and relationships as needed to prioritise your well-being and foster resilience in the face of life's challenges.

CHAPTER SEVEN: Conclusion

Reflections on the Journey through Grief

Grief is a complicated and intensely personal experience that is characterised by a wide range of feelings, difficulties, and realisations. Some thoughts on this voyage are as follows:

1. **Grief is Unique to Each Individual**: Grief is a highly individual experience, and no two journeys through grief are exactly alike. The way we grieve is influenced

by factors such as our relationship with the person we've lost, our personality, past experiences, and cultural or religious beliefs.

2. **It's Okay to Feel a Range of Emotions**: Grief encompasses a wide range of emotions, including sadness, anger, guilt, confusion, and even relief. It's important to allow ourselves to feel and express these emotions without judgement, as they are a natural part of the grieving process.

3. **Grief is Not Linear**: Grief doesn't follow a linear path or timeline, and

it's common for emotions to ebb and flow over time. There may be moments of intense sadness or longing, followed by periods of acceptance or even joy. It's important to be patient and compassionate with ourselves as we navigate the ups and downs of grief.

4. **Grief Can Bring Unexpected Growth**: While grief is undoubtedly painful, it can also be a catalyst for personal growth, self-discovery, and transformation. Through the process of grieving, we may gain insights into

ourselves, our relationships, and the nature of life and death. We may develop greater empathy, resilience, and appreciation for the preciousness of life.

5. **Healing is Possible, But It Takes Time**: Healing from grief is a gradual and ongoing process that unfolds at its own pace. While the pain of loss may never fully go away, it can become more manageable over time as we learn to integrate the loss into our lives and find ways to honour and remember our loved ones.

6. **Support is Essential**: Having a strong support network of friends, family, and professionals can make a significant difference in our ability to cope with grief. Sharing our feelings and experiences with others who understand can provide comfort, validation, and a sense of connection during difficult times.

7. **Finding Meaning Can Provide Comfort**: Finding meaning in our loss can be a source of comfort and solace as we navigate through grief. Whether it's through connecting with

others who have experienced similar losses, engaging in activities that honour our loved ones, or finding ways to make a positive impact in the world, finding meaning can help us find purpose and direction in pain.

8. **Honouring Our Loved Ones Matters**: Honouring the memory of our loved ones is an important part of the grieving process. Whether through creating memorials, participating in rituals, or carrying on their legacy in some way, finding ways to honour and remember our loved ones can help

keep their spirit alive in our hearts and minds.

9. **Self-Compassion is Key**: Above all, it's important to be kind, gentle, and compassionate with ourselves as we journey through grief. Grieving is hard work, and it's okay to take breaks, seek support, and practice self-care along the way. Remembering to treat ourselves with the same love and care that we would offer to a friend in need can help us navigate through grief with greater resilience and grace.

10. **There is Hope for the Future**: While grief may feel overwhelming at times, there is always hope for the future. With time, patience, and support, we can learn to carry our grief with us as we move forward, finding meaning, healing, and ultimately, a sense of peace and acceptance in our lives once again.

Encouragement for Readers to Continue their Healing Process

I want to inspire anyone who is going through the difficult process of getting over a loss or facing hardship.

1. **You are Stronger Than You Know**: Even on the darkest days, remember that you possess a strength within you that can withstand even the most difficult of trials. Trust in your resilience and your ability to overcome adversity, one step at a time.

2. **Healing is Not Linear**: Healing is a journey marked by ups and downs,

twists and turns. There will be days when you feel like you're making great progress, and others when you feel like you've taken a step back. Remember that this is all a natural part of the process and that every moment of struggle brings with it an opportunity for growth and renewal.

3. **Your Feelings are Valid**: Whatever emotions you're experiencing—whether it's sadness, anger, guilt, or something else entirely—know that your feelings are valid and deserving of

acknowledgement. Allow yourself the space to feel whatever you need to feel, without judgement or self-criticism.

4. **You Are Not Alone**: Even in your darkest moments, remember that you are not alone. Some people care about you, understand what you're going through, and are willing to support you every step of the way. Reach out to your support network, and let them help carry you through the tough times.

5. **Celebrate Your Progress**: Take a moment to recognise how far you've

come on your healing journey. Celebrate the small victories—the moments of joy, the instances of growth, the steps forward you've taken. Each one is a testament to your strength and resilience.

6. **Self-Care is Essential**: Remember to prioritise your well-being as you heal. Take time for self-care, whether it's through exercise, relaxation, spending time with loved ones, or engaging in activities you enjoy. Nurturing yourself is not selfish—it's necessary for your healing and growth.

7. **There is Hope for the Future**: Even amid pain and uncertainty, hold onto hope for the future. Know that brighter days lie ahead, filled with possibility, growth, and new beginnings. Keep moving forward with courage and determination, trusting that better days are on the horizon.

8. **Your Story Isn't Over Yet**: Your journey of healing is just one chapter in the larger story of your life. Embrace the challenges, the setbacks, and the triumphs, knowing that each experience shapes who you are and

prepares you for the chapters yet to come. Your story isn't over yet, and there are still many beautiful moments waiting to unfold.

Proceed, cherished peruser. Put one foot in front of the other, even if the route ahead appears intimidating. Keep reaching out for help, nurturing yourself with love and compassion, and believing in the potential of healing and rejuvenation. You are stronger than you think, and you can rediscover serenity, joy, and happiness.

A Glimmer of Hope

Once, there was a woman named Christine who faced the unimaginable pain of losing her husband, Jade, in a tragic accident. Christine and Jade had been inseparable since they were teenagers, building a life together filled with love, laughter, and shared dreams. When Jade was suddenly taken from her, Christine felt as though her entire world had shattered into a million pieces.

In the days and weeks that followed, Christine found herself drowning in grief. Every moment felt like an unbearable struggle, and she couldn't imagine how she would ever find the strength to go on without her beloved husband by her side. But as the days turned into weeks and the weeks into months, Christine began to find glimmers of hope amidst the darkness.

She found solace in the memories of their life together, cherishing every moment they had shared and holding onto the love they had for each other. She reached out to friends and family for support, allowing them to hold her up when she felt like she couldn't stand on her own. And most importantly, she allowed herself to feel the full depth of her emotions, embracing the pain of her loss rather than pushing it away.

As time passed, Christine began to find moments of peace and acceptance amidst her grief. She discovered that healing wasn't about forgetting her husband or moving on from her loss, but rather about learning to carry his memory with her as she continued to live her life. She found purpose in honouring his legacy, whether through volunteering, supporting causes he cared about, or simply living each day with the same kindness and compassion he had shown to others.

Through her journey of grief, Christine discovered a newfound resilience and strength within herself that she never knew she possessed. She realised that even in the face of unimaginable pain, she had the power to choose how she would respond—to choose love over despair, hope over fear, and life over loss.

And though Christine would always carry a piece of her husband's memory in her heart, she knew that she had the strength to face whatever challenges the future might hold. In the depths of her grief, she had found the courage to embrace life once again, knowing that love would always guide her through

even the darkest of days.